How to Mast

Positions

A Complete Guide to Boost Your Relationship Featuring
Positions from Easy to Advanced

America Sex Handbooks

professional before attempting any techniques outlined in this book.

By reading this document, the reader agrees that under no circumstances is the author responsible for any losses, direct or indirect, which are incurred as a result of the use of information contained within this document, including, but not limited to, — errors, omissions, or inaccuracies.

Table of contents

HOW TO DEEPLY CONNECT WITH YOUR PARTNERS

If we need more profundity and closeness and happiness in our connections, we will need to grow increasingly passionate association with our accomplices, our companions, our family, our colleagues. It's that straightforward and that difficult. Interfacing just through our playful feelings isn't sufficient—we additionally need to discover, and continue discovering, relationship-extending association through the entirety of our feelings. What's more, its absolutely impossible we can do this if we are not significantly close with our feelings.

Here are seven different ways to genuinely interface with your accomplice:

1. When you understand you're being responsive, state, "I'm being receptive."

How basic this sounds, but then how testing to incorporate—for the most part because of the disgrace we're on the edge of completely feeling as we become mindful of our reactivity.

What's more, when you've expressed that you're being receptive, STOP, regardless of how enticed you may be to proceed with your reactivity. Soften your tummy, inhale all the more profoundly, and hold up until you're prepared to state what you're feeling and that's it.

2. Figure out how to communicate your regret from your heart.

Try not to make due with shallow or genuinely level articulations. If you're not grieved, don't state you are—however if you've accomplished something that is harmed another and you feel terrible about this, and the words "I'm heartbroken" stall out in your throat, state that you're making some hard memories saying it. Such an admission will as a rule soften you enough to permit your regret a fitting voice.

3. If you're being guarded and know it, don't spare a moment to say as much.

Be your own informant. Try not to hang tight for the other to pressure you into owning up to your protectiveness. Also, don't slip into being cautious about being protective!

4. Try not to permit enthusiastic detachment to last any more drawn out than would normally be appropriate.

When you put some distance between the other, restore it as quickly as time permits. If you're remaining genuinely disengaged to rebuff the other, admit that at the earliest opportunity, paying little heed to how awkward that might be.

5. Never take steps to leave the relationship so as to get your own particular manner or to cause your accomplice to beseech you to remain.

If you want to be manipulative, say as much, instead of acting it out. Dangers are negative guarantees and are typically state of mind subordinate. If you truly need to leave a relationship, such needing will stay present regardless of how great, awful, or indifferent you feel.

6. Rather than utilizing sex to construct association, let sex be a completely typified articulation of effectively present association.

When you need to have intercourse when you are not associated with the other, direct your concentration toward your passionate state and take the necessary steps to bring that into your heart.

7. Remember that the more profound you plunge, the less you'll mind upsetting waves.

View your relationship as an ever-advancing experience, possibly extended by all that occurs, anyway upsetting. You may sting more as you develop, yet you'll mind less.

Following a monotonous day busy working, it's too simple even to consider coming home and thud down before the TV and space out. Remember about your relationship, however, and don't let your relationship get stale! These tips will assist you with feeling love regardless of whether you're exhausted from a taxing day. You'll build up a more profound association in your relationship in a matter of seconds!

1. Have significant discussions.

You can't feel an association with somebody if you can't generally converse with them. Do you feel a solid bind to the neighbor you gab about the climate with? It's farfetched. Be that as it may, if you halted and found out about their own life or convictions, you'd manufacture a relationship with them. It's actual—a few connections are easygoing, and simply require casual discussion. Yet, for the connections you esteem, ensure you set aside some effort to have a significant discussion and truly find a good pace individual.

2. Be available.

When you're with somebody, really be with them. Be available. Try not to be messaging on your telephone or focusing on something going on around you. Concentrate on who you're with and what they're stating. They'll see you're focusing and respond, which improves the relationship for both of you.

3. Give you give it a second thought.

When you're having these discussions, make sure it's understood you truly care. It's anything but difficult to profess to tune in and gesture in the correct spots, yet connections dependent on an association like this will feel empty and phony. Ensure you're put resources into the individual's life. They'll have the option to tell that you really care, and you'll feel more contributed and all the more cherishing towards them too.

4. Gain from your issues.

Try not to give a contradiction access a relationship progress into a ruinous contention. If you permit your feelings to go crazy and let a contention explode, it could cut off an association. Rather, keep your head level and work it out so there's a sensible trade off and all gatherings included need to proceed with the relationship.

5. Be available to different perspectives on affection.

Your accomplice may show love by doing little errands around the house for you, while you may wish they made amazing signals. Try not to reprove them for not indicating love the manner in which you need them to show love. Be available to different presentations of adoration. Discovering love in littler signals will assist you with seeing warmth and bliss in more things in life. In a matter of moments, you'll see that you show your affection in an assortment of ways, as well.

6. Give love.

Try not to hope to get love from everybody if you're not giving it out in equivalent measures. The more you give love and grace to individuals around you—companions, family, accomplices, associates, even outsiders openly— the more love and bliss you'll receive back consequently.

7. Focus on others' needs.

If you anticipate that others should thoroughly take care of you, you'll never feel any affection. It's critical to some of the time disregard getting your necessities met and see what individuals around you may require. Be benevolent and magnanimous to other people, and you'll get it back when you need it most.

8. Change your convictions about adoration and the world.

Try not to have a shut psyche when it comes to cherish and the world. If you're cut off, it will be more earnestly for affection to discover you. Keep a receptive outlook and an open heart. Love individuals paying little mind to what they do or what they look like. Keeping down adoration won't make anybody improve; it will simply transform you for the more terrible by making you put on a show of being egotistical and parsimonious.

9. Be grateful for everyone around you.

When you change your convictions about affection and the world, you'll find that it is so natural to be grateful for people around you. Everybody you experience in your regular daily existence is affecting you somehow or another, and you ought to be appreciative for them.

Value all your associates accomplish for you at work, what your family does at home, what your companions do to make you grin.

10. Love unequivocally.

Try not to adore somebody because they're doing admirably in school, or placing in extended periods grinding away. Try not to utilize love as a prize, and don't remove it as discipline. Love your loved ones a similar when they're having a decent day as when they're having a terrible day. If you love genuinely, you'll receive that adoration consequently and acknowledge the amount you truly need it.

THE SPIRITUALITY OF LOVE

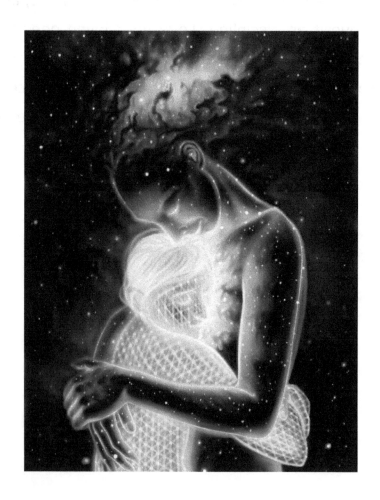

Individuals do insane things when it comes to adore. Some flee from home, others remain in a damaging relationship for the sake of affection, some quit their vocation because their adoration directed in this way, thus considerably more. The vast majority guarantee they are enamored however in actuality, they have no clue what the significance of genuine, profound love is. In certain connections, they are driven by fixation, envy, and terrorizing of their mate. They stalk their life partners wherever they go, they truly and intellectually misuse them, all for the sake of adoration. A few people go to the degree of ensuring their accomplices don't have any companions. That isn't a meaning of adoration; it is a fantasy of affection. The significance of profound love is when you can keep up your independence, in spite of the sentiment of enthusiasm. You can adore without applying any principles to one another. This is unequivocal love. It doesn't make a difference that your companion is revolting, shorter than you, or he snickers in a bothering way. You will adore that person the manner in which the person is. You will cherish all the blemishes the individual depicts and not reprimand them. Numerous individuals apply conditions in their connections, asserting they love one another. For example, you tell your life partner you love him when he gets you something. In otherworldly love, it resembles a spell that has been given occasion to feel qualms about you. You value your significant different as the individual in question is - no condition applies. You love him where it counts and you simply know it in your heart. If you ever wind up in such a circumstance, that is profound love. The following are a few rules to assist you with realizing you are genuinely enamored.

1.   You Communicate With Each Other With Ease

In each relationship, correspondence is the way to building a more grounded association. Couples must chat with other often and they should be in the same spot. If you can converse with your companion easily, he won't just tune in yet will likewise have sympathy for the current circumstance. You feel increased in value, you are regarded, and the greater part of all, no judgment is applied. Your companion underpins you completely in the entirety of your undertakings. In such cases, most couples appreciate what they have while it keeps going.

They appreciate each other's conversation and they normally search for private space to talk constantly. When one individual is talking, the other is listening acutely. No interferences, no thinking of different alternatives. You are both there for one another and bolster each other while being infatuated. An association in profound love is paid attention to very.

2. Uniformity Applies In Spiritual Love
A great many people don't have the foggiest idea about the meaning of uniformity in a relationship. It implies when two individuals interface and they chose to live respectively, jobs are characterized consequently. You can recognize each other's abilities and regard each other enough to let them do something amazing in your relationship. In each relationship, obligations come naturally. In profound love, you realize who is better at dealing with a specific part of your lives together. Trust applies in such a circumstance where you let your life partner start to lead the pack with no preference or judgment. This doesn't make either the individual in the couple lesser people, it just makes them more infatuated with one another.

3.You Are Attracted To Your Spouse

The vast majority don't have the foggiest idea what fascination implies. Some get pulled in to an individual because of their looks, how they dress, how rich they are, in addition to other things. Otherworldly love is when you need to interface with the individual, mind-wise, body-wise, and to the spirit. You need to be near the individual constantly. When you are as one, you feel an enthusiasm that you have never felt. It resembles an affection spell that has been provided reason to feel ambiguous about you. You are overcome with the energy and yet, you can remain rational. Your independence is as yet unblemished. Besides, there is a whole other world to life other than being diverted by desire.

4.   You Find Comfort in Each Other's Company

In profound love, there are no desires from one another, no sprucing up for the other. You simply present yourself as you seem to be. When you are enamored with one another, you feel that you can vanquish the world together. You don't see anything enormous under the sun. You experience happiness when you are as one and you don't scrutinize each other's dedication. Just you two comprehend your association. The manner in which you feel for one another has no simple definition. You simply feel content and your life will have an importance. In many connections, you will discover individuals addressing themselves. They don't believe their judgment and more often than not they rationalize to part. Others go through years seeking their accomplice and not making any genuine duty since they discover imperfections in each other. In otherworldly love, nothing of the sort applies. You love your companion as the individual in question seems to be. You value them for who they truly are. There are no butterflies or second-thinks about when you are as one.

5.   In Spiritual Love, There Is No Hurry

Society expects that when there is an association with the one you love, no time ought to be squandered, and you ought to rapidly make courses of action for your future together. Nonetheless, in otherworldly love, nothing of the sort is normal. Couples appreciate each other organization; they leave the destiny of their association to Mother Nature. You don't address if your life partner is the correct individual, if your companion going to be deeply inspired by another, etc. You heed your gut feelings that all will turn out fine and dandy. In profound love, you realize you are under this adoration spell together regardless of what occurs. The manner in which you see the world is the manner in which your mate sees it as well. You associate well with your sweetheart and offer energy.

6. Spiritual Love Promotes Growth

When you interface with somebody and you promise to live respectively, you hope to develop in all ways, particularly self-improvement. Your mate ought to be allowed to tell you your blemishes and you should take them decidedly. Tune in to your companion's recommendation. If somebody cherishes you, you ought not anticipate that the person in question should misdirect you. We can't accomplish self-improvement if our mates don't make some noise about our slip-ups. In profound love, you don't underestimate your mate nor do you consider him to be her as an apparatus to bring home the bacon. This is an extraordinary open door for you to encounter the genuine delight of being enamored.

7. Spiritual Love Does Not Let You Settle for Anything

As an individual, you are qualified for affection life, follow your interests, love a specific lifestyle, to be regarded and cherished. Your life partner ought to likewise esteem the things you love. The person in question ought not direct the manner in which you live. Your adoration ought to figure out how to join their necessities into yours. You should live in amicability and have the option to regard one another. These days, most duties are the inverse. Individuals settle for significantly less. They let their mates direct their method for living and have no common regard in the responsibility, all for the sake of "adoration".

8. Spiritual Love Enables You to Separate Fact from Feelings

In a responsibility resulting from affection, you will have a couple of battles about the years. Yet, that doesn't mean you have an awful relationship or your life partner loathes you. You will blow up at a portion of the remarks the person makes. Rather than misquoting one another, you ought to figure out how to work it out. Let your life partner clarify what the person in question implied.

9. In Spiritual Love, Couples Connect

Individuals in affection look at one another without flinching as they talk. Most customary couples talk for it. Some even talk with their back to their life partner. All things considered, couples who get each other are alright with confronting one another while taking. They can sit opposite one another at a table and speak with their eyes as it were. Who might not think they are under an affection spell? This shows how agreeable they are with one another and that certainty encompasses their adoration.

10. Spiritual Love Makes You Long For the Future

Each relationship differs from the others from numerous points of view. When two perfect partners love each other profoundly, they don't feel worn out on one another no problem at all. The fervor may blur with time, yet interest remains. You will cherish each other increasingly more with spending years. You are two people who have different qualities, however living respectively will empower both of you to investigate each other to the fullest as you age with time. Some case they began to look all starry eyed at from the start sight, however it requires significant investment and development to understand that you profoundly love your companion and that living without the person in question would be unfulfilling. Moreover, everyone might want a chance to develop old with their cherished one. These days, sweethearts settle for much less. They essentially need to profit by one another since they have no better choice. When they discover another person they feel an association with, they go separate ways as opposed to giving their adoration a possibility. Genuine affection requires some investment and tolerance. Indeed, even in the blessed writings of different religions, otherworldly love applies. To summarize everything, profound love is unqualified love that has no limits. It gives significance and significance to your life. Everybody wishes to encounter this sort of affection at one point in life. It is an awesome thing that can't be contrasted with some other inclination on the planet. It is elusive unequivocal love except if you practice some persistence. Couples who have a profound love are more joyful, they see one another, and they battle less. If you are in a profound love, give it your best since no one can really tell when it will end. Gain from one another and acknowledge what both of you have. You are more fortunate than others because you have encountered profound love and you know its definition.

SEX APPEAL

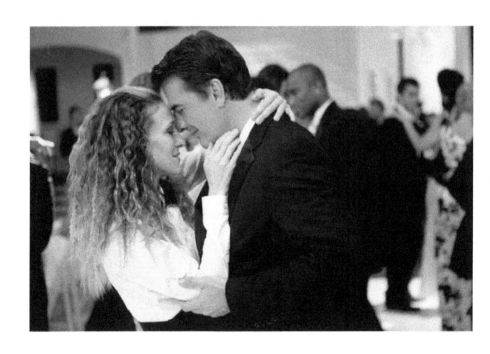

Have you at any point simply been so pulled in to somebody? The manner in which he talks, strolls, moves and his very quality make you need to be close to him and maybe do insidious things? He has sex claim, and you need him. To pull in him, you must engage in sexual relations advance, as well.

Yet, is sex offer only a unique little something you're brought into the world with? We don't think so! You can increment visual sex claim by focusing on your appearance. What's more, you can utilize non-verbal communication and the manner in which you act as a path how to engage in sexual relations claim if you realize what you're doing.

So read on to ace this easily overlooked detail known as sex claim!

Step by step instructions to

HAVE SEX APPEAL THROUGH BODY LANGUAGE

While we may state one thing with our mouths, we may be stating something else with our non-verbal communication. Stance, the manner in which we hold our arms and even the heading we face can impart a solid sign to somebody who realizes how to peruse non-verbal communication. For instance:

A grin is continually welcoming however be careful with counterfeit grins that don't arrive at the eyes.

Folding your arms or legs shows you're shut off. It's terrible if you're thinking about how to engage in sexual relations advance.

Right stance causes you to seem taller (and gives your chest a lift).

Squirming or skipping your advantage and down shows you're apprehensive.

Delicately contacting his arm is a simple method to be a tease. You can likewise lean in toward him to show you're intrigued. Become familiar with being a tease.

You'll will in general normally reflect his non-verbal communication if you like him. You can likewise do this intentionally, however don't impersonate everything he might do!

Look and face him to show you're focusing. Your eyes don't need to be spacey to show you're not so much put resources into the discussion.

Stroll with incredible and smooth advances. Know about your environment and have a confident nearness. Try not to fear the space you take up, which can make you recoil into yourself.

One way you can improve non-verbal communication is by focusing on what others do. How do certain and sexy individuals utilize their bodies? You can do that, as well!

Utilizing

YOUR APPEARANCE TO INCREASE SEX APPEAL

Let us prelude this by clarifying that there is no single size, shape or even hair shading that is sexy. Regardless of whether you fall outside the standard of what society thinks about sexy or beautiful, you've most likely pulled in the eye of somebody who believes you're saucy. Maybe you perceive how sexy you are, regardless of whether – or maybe because – you have a greater butt, you sport stretch imprints or your construct is somewhat more energetic than a few. You are sexy regardless!

My most impressive sex deceives and tips aren't on this site. If you need to get to them and give your darling back-angling, toe-twisting, shouting climaxes that will keep them sexually fixated on you, then you can get familiar with these mystery sex strategies in my private and careful bulletin. You'll additionally get familiar with the 5 perilous missteps that will destroy your sex life and relationship. Get it here.

Be that as it may, there are approaches to up your sex advance for a night out on the town if you truly need to dumbfound somebody.

Dress sexy: But what this implies will change contingent on your own style, body shape and solace level. Do you like pencil skirts? Pants? Plunging neck areas? Present day coats? Cowhide coats? Modern dresses? High-obeyed siphons? Knee-high boots? These things can engage in sexual relations claim, particularly if you pair them with intense certainty! There's no correct method to be sexy, and you can don't hesitate to disregard anything that's stylish if it doesn't fall into your usual range of familiarity. Then again, if you're typically a pants and-tee sort of young lady, which can be absolutely sexy, you may settle on something progressively female and coy when you go out. Individuals may be shocked, however don't let that prevent you from testing!

Regard your garments: All this implies is to keep your garments fit as a fiddle. Key upsetting in pants may be stylish and sexy, yet a monster gap in your pullover isn't!

Be particularly watchful with trim, work and weaved pieces, which are effortlessly damaged. While pressing isn't as famous as it once seemed to be, wrinkles are rarely sexy! Hang up your garments in the washroom while you shower, permitting the steam to discharge wrinkles.

Do your cosmetics: Again, this doesn't really mean you need to accomplish something outrageous, however a touch of establishment to try and out your skin tone, mascara to make your eyes pop and lip shine to cause to notice your sulk all expansion sex request. You can basically improve your normal highlights. What's more, if you're not happy with your aptitudes, head to your closest cosmetics counter to get some counsel and item suggestions. There are likewise a huge amount of magnificence Youtubers who make incredible video instructional exercises. If you're agreeable, you can observe progressively included cosmetics looks to truly wow individuals!

Treat your body right: No one anticipates that you should be great, however you can do various things to put your best face forward. Another approach to see this is your present propensities may be diminishing sex request.

Smoking cigarettes makes skin dull and ages you. Not getting enough rest gives you sacks under your eyes. An excess of liquor packs on the pounds, and insufficient water is awful for your skin and hair. So eat and drink well, get enough rest and work out. You'll look and feel much improved!

Smell wonderful: Have you at any point saw a person from over the room who looked sooo great? In any case, very close, you saw that he smelled terrible. Maybe he smoked, hadn't set aside the effort to tidy up after work or had poor oral cleanliness. Our feeling of smell is significant when it comes to sex advance, so you need to smell wonderful. Yet, it very well may be difficult to see how you smell by and by. This post has huge amounts of tips to guarantee you smell engaging.

Increment

SEX APPEAL THROUGH BEHAVIOR
Sex offer goes farther than what you look like! If you look great however have a character that leaves something to wanted, you may get laid a ton, yet you may wind up never-endingly single. Maybe you know somebody who falls into this class. All things considered, it's simpler to see someone else's deficiencies than our own.

Here are a couple of approaches to engage in sexual relations advance typically:

Be as agreeable as conceivable when conversing with individuals. Maybe you're anxious or bashful, which is alright because some folks like that! You may have tension or something different that makes it difficult to converse with anybody new, not to mention a potential date. This uncertainty is often evident to other people, and it can even cause everyone around you to feel ungainly. So you'll need to look over your discussion abilities and discover approaches to facilitate your tension – maybe a glass of wine!

Be certain. This binds in well to the past point. If you're not certain, it will in general show. Maybe you will in general put yourself down something over the top or think you'll be tenacious. More on that here. These attributes get old quick, in any case. Regardless of whether you're not so much sure about a circumstance, put a grin all over and make an effort not to allow it to appear. It's alright to chuckle about being somewhat anxious, however don't concentrate on it. Recall that others are lost in their own considerations, so it probably won't be obvious until you open your mouth and overplay it!

Try not to be a weakling! Folks really like when ladies have their own assessment. If you discover somebody who doesn't, consider why this may be and if you should kick him to the control. Have your own sentiments and don't be hesitant to go to bat for yourself. If you can differ pleasantly, it shows you're developed and astute!

Take a stab at something new. There's an adage about how you should have a go at something new consistently, and we concur! We comprehend this is actually quite difficult if you're on edge and ailing in certainty, yet you can get a lift once you effectively explore new territory. Indicating a person that you're not hesitant to have a go at something because you've never done it is one approach to engage in sexual relations bid! It doesn't need to be a serious deal, either. It could just request an insane dish from an eatery or seeing a film you don't think a lot about.

Stay positive. Nobody prefers a negative Nancy. It makes you less speaking to everybody whom you may meet. So stay cheerful. Try not to concentrate on the most exceedingly awful pieces of your life, despite the fact that you may be experiencing some difficult occasions. Nor would you like to speak awful about others. It makes you resemble a tattle!

Be fascinating. This may appear as though something you either are or aren't, yet that is not in reality obvious. If you have a comical inclination, you can make any story additionally intriguing. Be that as it may, if you keep yourself associated with interests and companions, read and stay refreshed with recent developments, you'll generally have something to discuss. When you can place some idea into what's happening around you and on the planet, you'll appear to be fascinating. That is unquestionably going to expand your sex claim!

One thing that a few people misconstrue about how to engage in sexual relations offer is that it's not tied in with being ostensibly sexual constantly. This can appear to be coarse or scaring to potential accomplices and everybody around you! It's smarter to indicate your sexuality as opposed to toss it in people groups' appearances. It looks truly senseless if you're attempting to profound throat an entire banana. Be that as it may, grinning and gently licking your lips is interesting without making others believe that you're making a decent attempt.

As you practice these aptitudes, they'll come the more no entire problem at all. Truly soon, you'll be flaunting your sex offer all over town. Recall not to conceal those one of a kind attributes that make you, you! That is a piece of engaging in sexual relations advance, as well!

FOREPLAY

Foreplay is viewed as any sexual movement before intercourse. All things considered, intercourse shouldn't be the great finale or even on the menu if you don't need. Incredible foreplay is bounty hot when done right.

For what reason is it significant?

Such a significant number of reasons! Foreplay triggers physiological and physical reactions that make sexual action pleasant and even conceivable.

Physiological

Truly, foreplay feels better, however it goes further than that. Participating in foreplay helps assemble passionate closeness that can cause you and your accomplice to feel increasingly associated all through the room.

Not in a relationship? Not an issue! Foreplay additionally brings down restraints, which can make sex more sultry among couples and virtual outsiders the same.

What's more, if stress has put a kibosh on your libido, a little foreplay may work.

Kissing, for instance, triggers an arrival of oxytocin, dopamine, and serotonin. This synthetic mixed drink brings down cortisol (stress hormone) levels, and expands sentiments of warmth, holding, and rapture.

Physical

Foreplay truly gets the juices streaming by expanding sexual excitement — which isn't to be mistaken for sexual want, however it can do that, as well.

Sexual excitement causes various physical reactions in your body, including:

- an expansion in your pulse, heartbeat, and circulatory strain
- widening of your veins, including your private parts
- more blood stream to the private parts, which causes the labia, clitoris, and penis to expand
- expanding of the bosoms and erect areolas
- greasing up of the vagina, which can make intercourse progressively agreeable and forestall torment

First of all: Foreplay implies different things to different individuals

As far as sex, foreplay is normally characterized as sensual incitement going before intercourse.

Remove intercourse from the condition and foreplay's characterized as an activity or conduct that goes before an occasion.

What that "occasion" involves may not appear to be identical to you as it does to another person — and that is flawlessly OK.

It doesn't need to prompt intercourse

Intercourse doesn't need to be the principle "course" or even on the menu if you don't need it to be.

It can really be the headliner!

Foreplay can stand its ground and be all you have to arrive at climax. Truly, look into has since a long time ago demonstrated that numerous individuals with vaginas don't climax with intercourse alone.

Along these lines, as long as there's assent, foreplay can be and incorporate anything you need.

You can even beginning well before things heat up

You need to begin some place, isn't that so? However, who says you should be without giving it much thought or even a similar space to begin?

If you need to draw out your play

If you realize you're getting together soon thereafter or even in a couple of days, you can utilize foreplay to kick the gathering off and prop it up. Here are a few plans to get you, well, began.

Leave a note

You don't should be inventive to make them go with a note!

A note left on their cushion or covered up in their duffel bag that suggests that you can hardly wait to take care of business later ought to work.

Sext

Messaging is simple peasy and should be possible on the fly.

A fast book mentioning to them what you will do to them or how hot it makes you when they [fill in the blanks] makes certain to get things mixing south of the fringe.

It likewise tells them you're contemplating them, and who doesn't adore that?

Get together for supper or beverages

Footsies under the table, a fast make out sesh in the bathroom or parking garage, or a nervy look at what you're wearing — or not wearing — under your garments.

These are only a couple of approaches to transform pre-fun supper or beverages into foreplay.

Pretend

Transform foreplay into a chance to experience your most stunning dreams by taking part in some pretend.

Claim to be outsiders set out toward a single night rendezvous when you meet for supper or beverages. Or on the other hand what about playing specialist and devious medical caretaker? You choose!

Kiss like you would not joke about this

Try not to send them off or welcome them with a peck. Rather, lock eyes, press your body against them, and kiss them long and profound.

Utilize your tongue and your hands and ensure you groan sufficiently only to get them excited for what's to come.

Reveal to them it's pre-game time

No should be bashful when your end game is to get them bare and do the unholiest of holies.

Let them know in as realistic a way as you can gather that there's nothing you need more than to get them hot and hard/wet and keep them that way the entire day and night long. Schwing!

If you need to start

Need something other than the wham bam? You can set the state of mind for foreplay and some other activity you need with the correct moves.

Light a few candles

There's not at all like candles to put things in place for all the sexy things.

Tea lights are modest, so stock up and light them all around any and each room you may get going in.

Did we notice how complimenting candlelight is on the skin?

Put some music on

We as a whole have a tune or two that contacts us somewhere down in our unique spot. Discover what theirs is, toss in yours for good measure, and make a playlist of others.

Barry White's "How about we Get it On" and Donna Summer's "Adoration to Love You" are two or three works of art. "Earned It" continuously is another mainstream track, and "Creature" by Nine Inch Nails is a hot one — and my own fave.

Move

Two bodies squeezed against one another and feeling each other's hot breath on your cheek as you influence to the cadence of sexy tunes. I rest my case.

Striptease

You needn't bother with a shaft or even incredible moves to do a striptease. Diminish the lights and take your garments off gradually with an articulation that shows no dread. Certainty can absolutely be faked, BTW.

Put out a sexual spread

Set up a cookout on the bed with a spread of some sexy treats that are made for sharing.

Delicious strawberries and fruits with some whipped cream and chocolate sauce for plunging are ideal for taking care of — and licking off — one another.

What's more, chocolate's a characteristic Spanish fly. Bon appétit!

Make out

Kick it ol' school and simply make out. Do it on the love seat, in the rear of a taxi, or squeezed facing the window.

If you're at the time

If you're as of now well on your way and feeling all the uncommon feels, it's the ideal opportunity for outercourse. Truly, that is a thing!

Here are a few things to attempt straightaway.

Back rub

The intensity of touch is genuine, and an exotic back rub does some incredible things for the body and brain. Light a few candles and get out the oil, or utilize a back rub flame that carries out twofold responsibility and can be Fifty Shades-esque.

Start at their feet and stir your way up, being certain to hit their erotic weight focuses and wait any place they need you to.

Erogenous zones

Your accomplice's body is a buffet of problem areas simply standing by to be contacted. Kiss, lick, and snack your way through the entirety of their erogenous zones.

Skin on skin

Dry bumping, it turns out, isn't only for horny adolescents. The sweet expectation of two bodies scouring against one another in different conditions of disrobe can't be beat.

Verbalize

Discussing what you need during sexy time doesn't simply function as foreplay; it likewise guarantees that you each get what you need and need in bed. Mention to them what turns you on and what you need to do to them.

Toys

There's something else entirely to sex toys than colossal cockerel formed dildos.

Vibrators of any shape and size can be utilized remotely on each erogenous zone you can consider.

There are likewise finger vibes and areola vibes you can use to take foreplay to another level.

A hot lathery shower

Hot wet skin and hands sliding over one another's bodies as you foam each other up with cleanser? Indeed please! A hot shower works, as well.

Tangible play

Not unreasonably such a lot of kissing and dry bumping won't stimulate the faculties, yet you can take it to the following level with a couple of props.

Blindfold your accomplice and bother them with different surfaces and temperatures with things like plumes, ice shapes, and your tongue.

Use things you as of now have that may feel great against the skin, or purchase a seduction unit on the web.

If you need to take things further

Prepared for your fundamental course? Make it an all-out blowout o' enjoyment with these thoughts.

Oral sex

Start away from the private parts and let your lips work their way down. Your mouth will do the majority of the work, yet don't let your hands get apathetic! Use them to stroke different pieces of their body while you delight them orally.

Make it hot. Try not to disregard the lesser known, yet quite pleasurable, bits while you're down there: the clitoral hood, which is the fold of skin over the highest point of the clit, and the frenulum, the little wrinkle of skin on the underside of the penis where the pole meets the head.

Protect it. Get some enhanced condoms and dental dams for safe oral sex. Yummy and sexually dependable!

Vaginal entrance

Vaginal entrance shouldn't be a definitive objective — it very well may be a stopover while in transit to whatever other sexual act that you're both into.

You can do it with fingers, sex toys and tie ons, or a penis or a mix.

Make it hot. Doing it doggy-style gives the infiltrating accomplice simple access to the accepting accomplice's G-spot. Furthermore, the view, well that is a reward.

Guard it. Lube is an unquestionable requirement regardless of what's doing the infiltrating. A warming lube will truly make entrance considerably more smoking.

Butt-centric entrance

Move slowly and appreciate some butt-centric play if you're both into it. Do it with your tongue, fingers, butt plugs, or a penis. Try not to hold back on the lube!

Make it hot. Doggy is by all accounts the position of the day! It gives the infiltrating accomplice simple access to the various parts that they should cherish on simultaneously, including the clit, penis, perineum, and prostate. Coming to these could get the accepting accomplice more like a butt-centric climax, as well.

Protect it. A hot foamy shower together prepares you for butt-centric play inside and out. It's likewise the ideal time to prod the opening with your tongue or a finger before going as far as possible.

Imagine a scenario where your accomplice doesn't appear to be keen on foreplay.

A few people simply don't appear to think about foreplay.

No doubt, being an apathetic or childish darling could be a piece of the issue, however it may very well additionally boil down to an absence of trust in their abilities or an absence of data about the how's and why's.

Discussing what you need in bed isn't in every case simple, particularly if you're stressed over harming or culpable your accomplice.

Here are a few hints to make it somewhat simpler:

Start on a positive note. Rather than referencing what they're not doing, start by mentioning to them what they do that feels better and how you need more. For instance: "I love it when you kiss my neck before we have intercourse. I could let you do that to me throughout the night."

Don't lay fault. Revealing to them your body's hankering something other than what's expected will go over much better than disclosing to them they're not fulfilling you.

Sharing time. Once in a while an individual needs some additional consolation. Whenever you embrace or kiss, hold them somewhat more and tenderly guide their hands along your body while revealing to them how great it feels. Viewing a video on tantric sex together may likewise give them a little bump the correct way, particularly if not needing foreplay has to do with an absence of skill.

Ask them what they need from you. Disclose to them how much turning them on turns you on. Follow with inquiring as to whether there's anything they need you to accomplish a greater amount of. It's an incredible method to open up the discourse so you can both offer what you need.

Disclose to them why it's imperative to you. You may need to lay everything on the table and cause them to comprehend why you need foreplay.

A few focuses that may merit referencing:

it encourages you get wetter/harder for sex

it encourages you climax or have more grounded climaxes

not every person gets excited at a similar pace and some need additional time than others

it encourages you feel nearer to them

it expands body familiarity with delight zones

The main concern

What sex and foreplay resemble to you doesn't have to agree with what you find in the media.

You don't need to follow a specific request or plan to appreciate either! It resembles having treat before supper — it'll be flavorful regardless of when you have it.

INTIMACY

What is sexual closeness? Sex is a demonstration shared among you and your mate that feels incredible and brings you closer. Closeness is a nearby enthusiastic bond among you and an accomplice. Unite the two and you have a profound association that will strengthen your marriage.

Being close methods something beyond getting physical with your accomplice. Having sexual closeness with your accomplice makes a profound enthusiastic association that adds to an additionally fulfilling sexual bond. Not every person will think that its simple to create sexual closeness and interface with their companion during sex. That is the reason we're taking a gander at 6 different ways you can extend your bond with your accomplice through sexual closeness.

What is sexual closeness?

When used to depict sentimental connections, closeness alludes to a nearby sexual association. Confiding in your life partner and feeling cherished, regarded, agreeable, and safe with them is an enormous piece of sexual closeness. Be that as it may, to characterize sexual closeness, we should have a more critical gander at what happens when accomplices approach.

Individuals let down their passionate watchmen during sex. Likewise, the arrival of the "nestle hormone" oxytocin triggers sentiments of connectedness that permits accomplices to be defenseless and build up trust with each other.

Having sexual closeness implies that you and your accomplice share a unique bond portrayed by a mutual sexy articulation. You see each other on a sexual level that has feeling behind it, rather than it simply being a physical demonstration.

Step by step instructions to associate sincerely during sex

What does being sexually associated mean? It's a physical and passionate bond with your mate. Figure out how to encourage this closeness by associating on a more profound level during sex. Numerous accomplices don't give a lot of consideration to sex and enthusiastic association however them two really supplement one another. Here are the absolute best tips on having a beautiful sexual association and how to make your sex life increasingly sentimental and significant.

1. Setting the stage

Do you need an all the more fulfilling physical and enthusiastic relationship with your accomplice? Who doesn't! One way you can interface more during sex is by making way for closeness. Some extraordinary thoughts for setting the disposition incorporate giving each other back rubs, put on a portion of your preferred erotic music, lighting candles, and clearing your calendars for sex and closeness.

If you're searching for a fast in and out, morning sex before work is your go-to. In any case, if you need to interface profoundly with your accomplice, pick a period where neither one of you will be intruded, for example, in the nights or on ends of the week.

Additionally, turn your telephone off. Nothing ruins sentiment in excess of a cellphone jingle going off out of sight to upset the enthusiastic association during sex.

2. Foreplay and development

One approach to interface during sex is to make a development. Bother your accomplice for the duration of the day with underhanded words, charged instant messages or messages, murmurs of romantic things and love, alongside cautious contacts to get them sincerely associated before the physical demonstration occurs. Working up to the minute will cause it to feel progressively extraordinary when it at last occurs. Feelings during sex run high and keeping up an association can take the experience to an entire different level inside and out. So the response to the ordinary inquiry – "how to be all the more sexually personal with your wife?" lies in sufficient measures of foreplay!

3. Keep in touch

It might feel clumsy from the outset, particularly if you're not used to looking affectionately at your accomplice, however keeping in touch with your mate during personal minutes not just encourages you associating sexually with your accomplice yet additionally assists with strengthening your bond.

This activity can cause you to feel open to your accomplice, which then cultivates sentiments of affection and trust. One investigation done by Kellerman, Lewis, and Laird uncovered that couples who kept in touch with each other detailed uplifted sentiments of adoration, enthusiasm, and general warmth toward their accomplices.

4. Talk during intercourse

What is sexual closeness? It's talking during sex. This doesn't mean you should begin having a discussion about what's for supper later.

There are two incredible roads for talking during sex that you can investigate with your accomplice. Initially, you can have a go at talking shrewd to each other. You can be as realistic or as held as you can imagine with this one. This an incredible method to release your restraints and interface with your words and dreams for getting physically involved with somebody.

You could likewise adopt an a lot better strategy and say romantic things to each other. Mention to your life partner what you like about what you are doing, reveal to them you love them, and state how close you feel to them.

Whatever words you pick, simply recollect that talking during sex is basically an approach to keep your consideration concentrated on each other during these sexually close minutes.

5. Participate in physical touch

How to make sex energetic? All things considered, when being private together don't be reluctant to contact the pieces of each other that aren't erogenous zones. Take a stab at stroking your better half's arms or run your hands through your wife's hair during the demonstration. This will assist you with interfacing on a passionate level and remind you to concentrate on each other during closeness.

6. Deal with one another's enthusiastic needs

One significant piece of a solid relationship is ensuring you are dealing with your life partner's passionate needs just as their physical ones which incorporates closeness and sex. Manufacture trust and show your accomplice regard to help make enthusiastic closeness.

Offer commendations and guarantee your accomplice of your adoration. Be fun loving with one another and have a normal night out on the town. The more associated you are outside of the room, the better your sex life will be. What's more, the less confused you will be about what is close sex. It's actually that straightforward!

7. Snuggle and kiss

Being personal when sex is an incredible method to encourage closeness. You can do this by kissing often. Kissing is an incredible method to construct strain and associate with your accomplice. Kissing is additionally appeared to expand serotonin, which causes you rest better, advance excitement, improve invulnerability, increment oxytocin and dopamine, and abatement stress.

Different approaches to build closeness is to snuggle after sex for a least two or three minutes, spoon before resting, and do a 6-second kiss each prior day going to work.

Sexual closeness happens when you have a sense of security, adored, and excited by your accomplice. There are numerous approaches to intensify your close association with your mate during personal sex. Set up a period where you will be separated from everyone else with your mate without interference, keep in touch during sex, and impart transparently about your physical and passionate needs. Doing this normally will prompt an additionally fulfilling sex life in your marriage.

Closeness. Individuals often mistake it for sex. In any case, individuals can be sexual without being private.

Single night rendezvous, companions with advantages, or sex without affection are instances of simply physical acts with no closeness included. They are what they are, however they don't encourage warmth, closeness or trust.

Closeness implies profoundly knowing someone else and feeling profoundly known. That doesn't occur in a discussion in a bar or during a stunning day at the sea shore or even on occasion during sex. It doesn't occur in the main many months of another and energizing relationship. It doesn't create when one individual sustains a relationship more than the other. No. Closeness, similar to fine wine sets aside effort to extend and smooth. It takes delicate dealing with and persistence by completely included. It takes the ability to commit errors and to excuse them for the sake of learning.

Closeness is the thing that a great many people long for yet not every person finds, or rather, makes. Why? Because closeness, genuine closeness with another person, can likewise be startling. Finding a good pace center of a relationship necessitates that the two individuals work through their dread. By visiting and returning to these regions, closeness develops and progresses after some time.

What Intimacy Involves:
Knowing: A really close connection tells the two individuals on the most profound level who they each genuinely are. They have investigated each other's spirit and discovered what something they esteem and acknowledge such a lot of that it can withstand the unavoidable differences that exist between any two people.

Acknowledgment: Neither individual wants to change the other or to change themselves in basic manners. Gracious truly, minor changes consistently happen when individuals suit each other to live respectively. Yet, neither individual from the couple thinks to oneself, "Well — with time, I'll get that person to change what their identity is."

Valuation for differences: Both comprehend that they don't should be totally the equivalent to be close. Actually, some portion of the enjoyment of connections is the disclosure of differences and thankfulness for one another's uniqueness. Finding out about one another's perspectives is viewed as a chance to grow their universes.

Wellbeing: True closeness happens when the two individuals have a sense of security enough to be powerless. There is support for one another's shortcomings and festivity of one another's qualities. The couple has conceded to a meaning of devotion and both have a sense of safety that the other won't abuse that understanding.

Sympathetic critical thinking: Elephants don't come to remain in the "room" of the relationship. Issues are stood up to by the two individuals with affection, empathy and an ability to draw in with whatever issues have come up. The two work to be on a similar group, taking care of an issue, instead of on different groups contending with one another.

Enthusiastic association: Intimacy develops when individuals remain genuinely associated, in any event, when there are issues to explain. It doesn't require that either individual tread lightly or retain what they truly think so as to remain associated.

The most effective method to Nurture Intimacy:

Pick shrewdly: The principal rule for having a close connection is to pick admirably in any case. If being in the relationship with your beau/sweetheart necessitates that you surrender who you truly are, that you generally oblige, or that you roll out crucial improvements to be satisfactory, this individual isn't for you. Much all the more telling is if your accomplice normally charges, faults or bothers you or necessitates that you not remain near different companions. Cut your misfortunes. Get out. Make yourself accessible for somebody who will respect and value you and bolster you for what your identity is.

Show yourselves: As another relationship develops, bit by bit demonstrate yourselves to one another – both the most appealing and the not all that alluring highlights of what your identity is. Be happy to uncover your center convictions, qualities and thoughts to find different's responses. Alternate extremes may at first pull in however they are likewise often the seeds of disappointment as a relationship advances after some time. Investigate your differences and choose if they are fascinating and energizing or major issues. Ensure that your differences don't damage fundamental beliefs for either individual.

Draw a circle: Intimacy necessitates that your relationship with one another is by one way or another different from your associations with every other person. Numerous couples draw the limit around their sexual selectiveness. Others characterize their closeness in different manners. Whatever your choice about devotion, there should be something you both concur is the center of what makes your relationship exceptional, valuable, and extraordinary from all others. Both concur that limit is critical to the point that disregarding it would shake the very establishment of your couple-ness.

Create passionate care: Emotions aren't fortunate or unfortunate. Be that as it may, how we express them can either improve or harm closeness. It's inescapable that every one of you will feel outrage, hurt or disillusionment on occasion, maybe even commonly. Closeness requires learning approaches to communicate those sentiments that are neither threatening nor removing. Work together to find approaches to quiet extreme emotions as opposed to becoming involved with them. Consent to chip away at finding and tending to the base of issues as opposed to detonating or pulling back.

Grasp struggle: Yes, grasp it. Overlooking clash once in a while fills in as a way to closeness. Whatever the contention was about just goes underground, putrefies, and inevitably turns out in ugly and often antagonistic ways. Strife is a sign that there is an issue that should be illuminated. Closeness requires confronting issues with fortitude and with the confidence that the relationship is a higher priority than whatever emergency is going on at the time.

Be the individual you need your accomplice to be: It's anything but difficult to need another person to be understanding, sympathetic, devoted, giving and liberal. It's not all that simple to do it. Closeness necessitates that we do our absolute best to be somebody worth getting physically involved with. It's not important to be flawless at it. It is important to put forth a valiant effort and to be available to criticism when we come up short.

EASY SEX POSITION

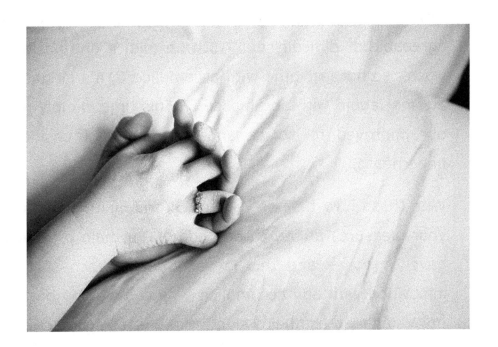

If there's a small piece of you thinking "ouch" during sex, then it's a great opportunity to return to your room methodology. Sex ought to never be awkward... aside from possibly in that divertingly ungainly way.

Regardless of whether position A worked for your past accomplice, your new S.O. will be evidently different. How their own taste lines up with yours will decide agreeable or difficult sex. Truth be told, if one position wasn't so hot last time with accomplice C, it's alright to attempt again with accomplice D. This time, simply join our improved for-solace and-fulfillment sex positions underneath.

With these how-tos, we've kept clitoral incitement (and your pleasure) at the cutting edge. The main prep you have to do — and this is valid before each sort of infiltration with any accomplice — is convey and grease up! Vaginal grease helps significantly lessen contact and inconvenience (and it's flawlessly alright to utilize lube) and prepares for satisfying sex.

Sizzling preacher
Relinquish any old recollections of those blameless occasions when fairly cadenced here and there was all

you thought about sex. Rather, make another experience of the exemplary minister. Instead of broadening your legs, have your accomplice's legs straddle your body, allowing for shared genital contacting. This works incredible because it isn't subject to estimate yet on the association you and your accomplice have.

Sitting on pad top

Take your preferred pad, and spot it underneath your pelvis for expanded help. Curve your knees, bring your pelvis upward, and spread your legs sufficiently separated to take into consideration pushing. What's fabulous about this position is that it permits you to control the profundity of infiltration and advances clitoral incitement.

Riding into the nightfall

Take control and jump on top. This position is perfect for some comfortable occasions because it takes into consideration personal kissing and eye staring, and allows you to make the beat you most appreciate. Not exclusively will you have the option to situate your clitoris just as you would prefer and increment sexual joy, yet you can likewise shake your pelvis to and fro to make an agreeable mood.

Incline toward me

Discover a divider or table to incline toward. Face one another and pick who will hold each other's butts, and snare their leg around the other individual's leg for help. Animate one another, by scouring your clitoris against your accomplice's private parts, and afterward make an agreeable musicality whereby you're ready to draw your body nearer or away.

Side nestle

You can either confront one another, or position yourself to allow section from behind. If you're confronting your accomplice, you can take rule of your sex toy or the penis shaft and make the point and push you want. In the back section position, utilize your rear end to control the speed and have your accomplice stay still, while you move at your own pace and control the profundity.

The couple

Pair your preferred situation with self-joy by fusing the manner in which you like to feel great at the same time. If you're utilized to self-animating your clitoris while lying on your back, with or without a sex toy, then do only that while welcoming your accomplice to contact your bosoms or kiss you. Making this pair sensation can be explosive.

The bunny

Who said that sex toys are just for solo play? Residue off your preferred vibrator and demonstrate it to your accomplice. Plan to utilize it next time by legitimately applying clitoral incitement while you explore different avenues regarding different positions.

Utilize the different vibration settings to expand your pleasure or bother each other. Take a stab at holding off on climaxing until you can't keep down. The most significant thing, generally, when including another sex toy, is that you both convey about everything without exception — particularly on what feels great to one another.

The blacklist

If you've had a go at everything, you're despite everything encountering torment — particularly with infiltration — then it's a great opportunity to blacklist entrance for a tad. To substitute, practice sensate center activities. Maintain the emphasis on developing sexy touch, sexual back rub, and delight rather than execution.

To flavor things up throughout this break, you could check out 69. Just, go on your back and have your significant other's mouth face your private parts, while you discover your mouth to theirs. Set aside the effort to appreciate investigating one another.

When you're an amateur, sex can feel truly overpowering, so there's no disgrace in discovering some simple sex positions to assist you with finding your feet. It requires some investment to realize what you like, what your accomplice loves, and even exactly how things fit together once in a while. What's more, don't kick me off on how to manage your hands if you're on top. I may never get that right. I've simply kind of surrendered.

If you don't know where to begin, simply recollect that one of the most significant things is to back off and permit yourself to unwind. "Perhaps the best activity when your accomplice has constrained sexual experience is to focus on your pace," Tristan Weedmark, worldwide energy represetative for We-Vibe tells Bustle. "There's no motivation to hurry into something in bed that may incite uneasiness. Peruse your accomplice's non-verbal communication and remain aware of how rapidly you're moving." And if you're both new to it that is no issue—you can find what you like together.

So move slowly with places that won't be excessively testing, moves where you can concentrate on making sense of things, and places that vibe cozy, protected and associated. Here are some incredible ones to attempt if you're a novice:

Vis-à-vis

Step by step instructions to Do It: Laying on your sides and confronting one another, move marginally higher up on the bed—so your hips are over your partner's. Fold your top leg over them and guide them within you. Lube can help if it's an unbalanced fit.

Why It's Great For Beginners: If you're new, you will be on top of your accomplice to ensure you're both agreeable. This is a cozy position that you can unwind into — with profound entrance.

Teacher

Instructions to Do It: If you start in minister, have your accomplice move their hips higher up the bed while you fold your legs over them. This will give you much more incitement than conventional evangelist.

Why It's Great For Beginners: Missionary is an incredible go-to for novices, however this variety is a superior situation for climax. In addition, you're both in an agreeable situation to simply concentrate on one another and ensure you're both getting what you need.

On Top (Modified)

Step by step instructions to Do It: Have your accomplice incline toward the divider or a sofa while you straddle them and drop down. For significantly more closeness, they can twist their knees so they're helping prop you up.

Why It's Great For Beginners: On top is an extraordinary position, however a few ladies feel somewhat uncovered or awkward — particularly when they're unpracticed. This permits you to be in charge, however with an increasingly cozy and associated alternative.

Doggy

Step by step instructions to Do It: Rest on all fours and spread your legs so your accomplice can bow behind you. You may require your legs further separated or closer together, contingent upon your stature differences.

Why It's Great For Beginners: Even however you're new, you may like greater force. This position lets you try different things with more profound infiltration and leaves a hand free for clit play.

Modified Doggy

The most effective method to Do It: Either change from doggy style down onto your elbows, or start by laying on your stomach. A pad under your hips can assist you with finding the correct edge.

Why It's Great For Beginners: If doggy is unreasonably exceptional for you, this is gentler—yet similarly as sexy. It's likewise extraordinary for any murmuring or filthy talk you need to attempt.

Spooning

The most effective method to Do It: Lay in the spooning position with your hips over your partner's. Lift your top leg somewhat so your accomplice can enter you. If it's a cumbersome fit, attempt some lube.

Why It's Great For Beginners: Another choice for G-spot incitement, yet this is the most agreeable one. When you get the fit right, you can simply appreciate it.

Cowgirl

Step by step instructions to Do It: Once you're feeling progressively good and more certain, you can go for full cowgirl. Straddle your accomplice and guide them inside you. You can generally utilize your hands to help balance.

Why It's Great For Beginners: You can lean forward, back, bob, pound, and so forth. It's an incredible situation for a learner to realize what they like, and it offers extraordinary perspectives and eye to eye connection.

If you're an amateur, there's no disgrace in taking as much time as is needed to make sense of what you like. Move slow and follow what feels better — there's bounty to browse.

INTERMEDIATE SEX POSITIONS

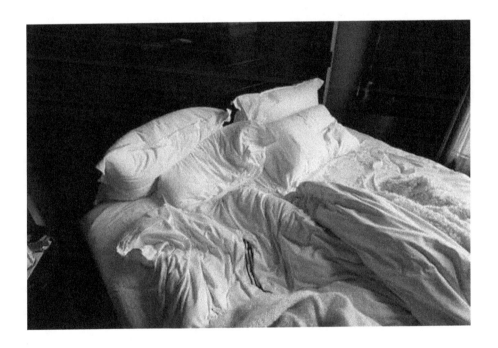

Toward the day's end, sex is much the same as some other game or performing artistry:

The conclusive outcome is just worth the vitality and practice you put into it.

Sex can be out and out enticing, or an all out nap fest — and a great deal of it has to do with the measure of exertion that you and the lady you're with placed into it.

So if you're prepared to change it up a bit, and zest up your sex life... it can mean the difference between exhausting, unremarkable sex, and completely amazing sex.

(I don't think about you, yet I'll take the last mentioned — and as quite a bit of it as I can get, if you don't mind)

Sex ought to be something you and your accomplice ceaselessly gain from and improve, so as to keep it crisp, energizing, and pleasant.

So whether you're new to engaging in sexual relations...

Searching for further developed, test, or plain different sex positions...

Or on the other hand searching for different sex positions to drive her wild...

You've gone to the opportune spot.

Amateur Vs. Transitional Vs. Propelled: How To Choose the Right Positions For You

Right now, going to walk you through the best different sex positions for:

Amateurs hoping to ace fundamental sex moves...

Experienced individuals hoping to analyze or get familiar with some new deceives...

Those keen on discovering moves that drive her wild and take her over the edge...

Also, significantly more. I'll show you the 5 best moves for every class, experience what makes them so hot, and disclose how to give them a shot.

In any case, before we start, you may be pondering:

"How would I know if I'm a tenderfoot or further developed?"

Also, at last, I can't answer that — no one but you can genuinely respond to that question for yourself.

Be that as it may, if you aren't sure, my suggestion is to skim through the "Apprentice" positions and proceed onward to the accompanying segments once you feel acquainted with those.

While these moves probably won't work superbly for everybody, there are varieties you can give it a shot and edge alteration suggestions that will assist you with idealizing each position.

Have you previously aced the fundamentals... ?

Or on the other hand perhaps you're simply searching for to a greater degree a test in bed... ?

Maybe you and your better half are needing to explore, yet you don't know precisely where to begin.

These 5 positions will be extraordinary venturing stones into your experimentation with sex. Additionally, huge numbers of them can be performed with props or subjugation methods to kick it up an indent truly.

Doggy Style
different-sex-positions-doggy-style

This is an extraordinary situation to evaluate when you first beginning spicing things up...

If you've never attempted this cherished position or if you're hoping to get progressively exploratory, Doggy Style is the ideal spot to begin.

It's an incredible prologue to more unpleasant sex and can be strongly pleasurable for both you and the lady you're with.

To consummate this position, have her bow down on the bed, then lower her chest area so she's on all fours.

Bow or set down behind her and enter her from behind.

Additionally, remember that you will likely need to play with the point after you enter her.

For instance, a 90-degree (opposite) edge of section probably won't feel astounding for her...

Be that as it may, utilizing pads or having her let her head down could help twist her body with the goal that you're entering from an edge she cherishes.

If you've just aced this position or you're hoping to kick things up a score, then Doggy Style is likewise an extraordinary method to begin trying different things with butt-centric sex.

Start with toys first, and change the edge until both of you are agreeable enough to pull out all the stops.

For an additional tad of wrinkle, have a go at riding her while pulling her hair or secures her.

(As a lady, I can reveal to you that the vast majority of us need you to be truly unpleasant with us in bed... here are 3 different ways to do it I guarantee she'll adore.)

Spread Eagle
This is an incredible situation to investigate some light BDSM...

If you're truly hoping to flavor up your sex life, there's nothing better than a move that requires some minor subjugation.

The Spread Eagle is an unfathomable situation for anybody keen on dallying with BDSM or simply searching for some additional enjoyment in bed.

To consummate this position, have her rests on her back. Next, have her lift her legs and arms open to question.

If you'd like, you can make it so her legs and arms contact.

What's more, to be significantly kinkier, you can tie her legs and her arms together. Ensure the bunch is tight, yet not very tight to remove her flow.

At last, enter her from above (like Missionary).

This places you in unlimited authority of the circumstance, which is perfect if you're hoping to play with Dominant/Submissive jobs.

Regardless of whether you aren't into BDSM, this position can be amazingly exciting, insofar as there is finished trust among you and your accomplice.

Reverse Cowgirl
Bid farewell to preacher with the Reverse Cowgirl

Overjoyed up, rancher!

Put her in the driver's seat with this unbelievable position.

This variety of Girl on Top offers her more authority over the circumstance, while likewise permitting you to loosen up additional. Furthermore, you get an extraordinary view while you're doing it. Falsehood level on your back or at an edge and have her straddle you with the goal that she's confronting your feet. She would then be able to utilize her thighs to swivel and bob here and there.

To make it somewhat more extraordinary and to give her some more influence, twist your knees so she can utilize them to help lift her body here and there.

What's more, if you need to take this position considerably further, have her secure you so you can't do anything aside from lay back and appreciate the ride.

Inclined Doggy Style
If you have stairs you're certainly going to need to evaluate this position...

Do you want to try different things with certain edges? This position is ideal for you.

It's one of the most creative modifications to customary Doggy Style and may be exactly what you have to flavor up your sex life.

You'll require stairs to get this going, and it's additionally an extraordinary situation for both vaginal and butt-centric sex — I'll allow you to choose.

To pull it off, have the lady you're with bow on a stair and let her slender forward with her chest area so she's laying on the means over her legs.

Then you do likewise, with the exception of your chest area will lay on hers as you enter her from behind.

It's perhaps the most ideal approaches to make sense of what points drive both of you wild and can be the ideal "entryway tranquilize" to begin trying different things with sex in unusual spots.

Wet and Wild
Evaluate this situation for some additional enjoyment in the shower...

You don't need to consolidate shiny new moves into the room to test — rather, have a go at changing your condition.

Shower sex can be a great deal of fun (insofar as you're cautious), so if you're hoping to switch up your sex normal, simply include water.

To be effective at shower sex, ensure you have an amazing silicone-based lube for her and something solid for you to clutch.

You can attempt a standing Doggy Style position where she twists around, or you could likewise take a stab at standing vis-à-vis while you enter her (twist her leg for help).

Trying different things with sex is an enjoyment part of any solid relationship, so don't let the positions accomplish all the work for you.

Take a stab at consolidating messy talk...

Sex toys...

Servitude...

Or on the other hand different props that you both concur will truly help push things to the following super-sexy level.

While sex is typically a ton of good times for the vast majority of us women...

It can in any case be extremely difficult to really have a climax during the deed (regardless of whether what you're doing feels incredibly great).

Nonetheless, while climaxing during sex can be a genuine test for most ladies — it's unquestionably not feasible.

(Like did you realize her climax is 80% almost certain if you can do this to her? It's so cracking simple as well.)

Perhaps the most straightforward ways for a lady to climax through intercourse is by putting her in the driver's seat. Along these lines, she can animate her body the manner in which she needs.

Obviously, there are likewise ways for you to control her developments while additionally taking her breath away.

So if you need to do all that you can to give her the sexual delight she hungers for, have a go at including (at least one) of these sex positions to your arms stockpile.

The Fusion
This Fusion position is extraordinary for increasingly extreme climaxes...

This position is somewhat more entangled to pull off, yet it's so worth the exertion.

It offers better development control for her while furnishing you with the best view in the house. ☺

To consummate this position, sit on the bed with your legs spread. Then recline and prop yourself up utilizing the palms of your hands.

From that point, have her sit confronting you between your legs, and prop her decisive advantages over your shoulders. She'll likewise be reclining somewhat and supporting her weight with her palms.

This position permits her to go all over or around and around, giving quicker and increasingly serious climaxes for both of you.

The Waterfall
Evaluate this Waterfall strategy for a totally different edge and more profound infiltration...

This position doesn't occur in the shower — rather, it's named after the manner in which it looks.

In addition to the fact that it provides better power over developments for her, yet it additionally guarantees you have probably the best climax of your life.

Give it a shot by laying level on your back (at the foot of the bed).

Gradually slide your take and back off of the bed with the goal that your head and shoulders are on the floor.

Now, your body will be curved in a sort of cascade shape. Next, have her sit on you — from that point, she can squeeze her heels against the edge of the bed and crush and down, moving her hips around and around.

The genuine mystery to this stunt is that the blood in your body is going to race to your head, making your climax considerably more extraordinary than you at any point thought conceivable.

It's additionally phenomenal for her because she can prod you while developing to her own climax.

Lowered Reverse Cowgirl
Evaluate this changed form of Reverse Cowgirl... Like Reverse Cowgirl, this move keeps the lady in charge everything being equal.

What makes it different here is that her body will be in a superior situation to really explore her developments all the more decisively — this builds her odds of arriving at climax significantly.

To pull off this position, get into the standard Reverse Cowgirl position.

From that point, have her let herself down to your legs or feet, and she can utilize the palms of her hands and her knees to help bolster her body.

This will offer her better command over her developments, permitting her to hit quite a few spots.

Pinball Wizard
Make her climax hard with the Pinball Wizard move..

Did you experience childhood with arcade games? Pinball, maybe?

All things considered, consider this the "grown-up" variant of pinball.

This position gives you control of the circumstance and furthermore makes it simpler to bring the lady you're with to climax.

What's better, it should likewise be possible as unpleasant (or "vanilla") as you need and can be modified in a couple of different ways.

To consummate this position, stoop down on the bed and have her lay before you.

Lift her advantages and grasp her thighs to help push in and out.

You can modify this somewhat by having her ribbon her lower legs around your neck or over your shoulders.

This hot position feels naughtier than most... but on the other hand it's an incredible method to give her a simple climax (the chances of a lady having a climax are expanded whenever her legs are noticeable all around).

Magic Mountain
Make sex into an enjoyment ride with this Magic Mountain move...

The "Enchantment Mountain" doesn't simply stable like an enjoyment ride at an entertainment mecca... it likewise feels astonishing.

It makes it similarly simple for both you and the lady you're with to control your developments — and what's more, it makes it route simpler for her to get done with during sex.

Put a pile of cushions on the floor. Have the lady you're with hang over the pads and "unwind" into them.

Her back should normally curve.

You need to lay on her back so your chest is "stuck" to her. Your arms ought to be on hers.

Then enter her from behind, much the same as doggie style.

You can now securely go "full scale" with your pushes, since she has a lot of cushioning.

Be that as it may, it likewise gives her an expanded feeling of association and skin-to-skin contact.

The best part about this move is that there's a mutual feeling of sexual control.

By the day's end, sex ought to be a good time for both you and the lady you're with... and these positions ought to absolutely assist you with arriving.

In any case, I have to admit — there is one more thing you can do to ensure you're really great she's at any point had.

ADVANCED SEX POSITIONS

Sex resembles frozen yogurt; we as a whole have our preferred flavor. When we've discovered the one that that fulfills us without fail, we stay with it. Hello, why fix anything if it's not broken? Yet, let's be honest, treats 'n' cream after a long time after night will have even the most committed client desiring another spoonful to appreciate.

Regardless of whether we're discussing tidbits or sex positions, it's acceptable to attempt new things. As per an ongoing sex study, the best indicator of long haul sexual fulfillment for couples was an ability to take a stab at something new, and sex positions were at the highest priority on the rundown.

Indeed, while you may have aced preacher and doggy-style back in your 20s, there's in no way like the rush of playing with some wild moves together. Attempting new, progressively brave sex positions won't just assist you with enduring longer, yet will likewise stretch out the excursion to peak, making those last minutes such a great amount of better for you both.

Be cautious, however — these positions are not for fledglings.

Feline (COITAL ALIGNMENT TECHNIQUE)

For ladies that experience difficulty arriving at climax through intercourse alone, the Coital Alignment Technique (otherwise called the CAT position) can be The One. What's more, what man wouldn't like to be the person who gets her there?

To nail the CAT position, start off in preacher and, after infiltration, slide your pelvis a couple of inches higher than expected. Keep your body level against hers and as opposed to moving in and out, concoct and down — the key here is to be pelvis-to-pelvis so the base of your penis can invigorate your accomplice's clitoris. She should fold her legs over you, either keeping her hips still or turning them for more noteworthy contact. If you're experiencing difficulty hitting the spot, have a go at setting a cushion under her butt or making a roundabout movement with your hips. Snatching the headboard and consolidating pulls with hip pushes assists with your point and lets you infiltrate her more profound. To really open this current position's latent capacity, reach your pelvic bone as the consistent, shaking movement brings you both to an incredible peak. Go on, rock her reality.

The sitting v

Despite the fact that the Sitting V is an entirely clear situation for men, it requires a specific measure of adaptability from your accomplice. What amount? Consider this: if she can't contact her toes in a forward overlap, it probably won't be the correct decision. To pull it off, have your sweetheart sit on a high seat or ledge confronting you, while you face her with your feet spread separated. Modify the separation until your pelvis adjusts flawlessly with hers before having her place her lower legs over your shoulders, moving her body into an 'Angular' shape against you. She would then be able to recline, utilizing the divider or her arms as help, or pull herself closer to you by folding her arms over your neck (Although this alternative builds the stretch on her hamstrings)... If you need to help make the position increasingly agreeable for her, have a go at supporting her middle with your hands around her back.

This position permits you to infiltrate your accomplice profoundly and control the beat and profundity of your developments, letting you set the tone to the peak. The capacity for ground-breaking pushing, joined easily of execution, can make this a seriously animating posture.

The scissors

Not simply held for young lady on-young lady activity, scissoring can truly hit the spot for hetero couples too. Begin sitting up on a delicate surface with your legs collapsed in a topsy turvy "V" while she lays on her side with her legs open and knees somewhat twisted; your lower parts should meet an a nearly right point. Spot your upper leg over her lower leg and your lower leg underneath hers, then shift sufficiently close to enter her. In spite of the fact that it might be dubious to locate the ideal situation from the start, when you get it, the laid-back yet extreme incitement will keep you and your darling returning for additional.

The Scissors probably won't permit a lot of scope of movement, yet don't be debilitated — there's a lot of joy to be had for all! The situating of your entwined legs gives your accomplice persistent clitoral incitement, while the shallow pushes energize the nerve endings on the leader of your penis, taking into consideration an electrifying form to climax.

Face-sitting

Not unreasonably you need a reason to go downtown, however face-sitting presents an agreeable, low-sway approach to give your woman unadulterated euphoria. If you wind up requiring a minute to regain some composure between positions, or are feeling — ahem — over-animated, lay back and put the attention on the main thing: her pleasure. Have your accomplice straddle your head, being certain to leave you a couple of crawls of breathing room, before she settles in and you get down to business. Odds are she'll require something to clutch, since you'll be doing such a great job causing her to squirm with joy. A divider or bedpost proves to be useful for balance, while tucking her calves under your shoulders includes additional steadiness.

This posture is useful for those as yet culminating their tongue strategy, as it permits the face-sitter to control the position and force more definitely than if she was laying on her back. Also, most definitely... If the view from this edge wasn't sufficient to make you go, her butt and hips are in simple reach for a crush of enjoyment.

Sideways 69

It resembles I generally state, once in a while you have to give a little to get a bit. However, there's definitely no explanation that you can't give and get at the equivalent, isn't that so? That is the reason 69 is such a fan-most loved in the room, because it permits us to furnish a band together with consistent delight without sacrificing our very own moment. Also, when you turn 69 on its side, you can give for such a long time you could conceivably be blessed sainthood.

Start by laying on your side confronting your accomplice, with your head toward her feet and the other way around. Next, twist your top leg to frame a triangle, with your knee pointing at the roof, putting the top foot level on the bed and supporting yourself on your elbow for balance. Contingent upon your stature and size, you may need to modify the good ways from your accomplice to advance access to their genitals. Despite the fact that it's substantially less famous than customary 69, this sideways variety takes out potential neck-hurts and opens up your hands to participate in the pleasuring, in addition to it's often increasingly agreeable and less unbalanced to hold for an all-inclusive timeframe. Cheerful 69ing!

Cascade

If you're similar to most couples, there are numerous evenings you likely would prefer not to get off the lounge chair — so why not get off on the sofa? The Waterfall is a minor departure from the famous Cowgirl position, yet sneaks up all of a sudden. Start by laying on the lounge chair or bed with your head close to the edge and your young lady on you, however as opposed to riding you from her knees, she'll have to recline and shift her weight to her feet. When she has the position down, crawl toward the edge of the bed or lounge chair, letting your head and shoulders slide off onto the ground while your hips stay raised. If you're on a lounge chair, wrap your legs over the rear of the situate or basically let your knees fall open. From here, your accomplice has unlimited oversight over the speed, profundity and force of her gyrations, also a free hand to use as she wishes — clitoral incitement, anybody?

There are a few different ways to execute this posture: You can either utilize it as a scaffold while working to climax, or moving into it directly before the enormous finale. In any case, this position will make the blood hurry to your head (and your other head) for a dangerous peak.

(Presently you'll comprehend why it's known as the Waterfall).

G-SPOT SEX POSITIONS

If a lady's life structures were Disney World (not to make Disney unusual or anything...), her clitoris would be the Magic Kingdom—the headliner where all the enjoyment and firecrackers occur. What's more, her G-detect, a little hotspot more profound inside her, ahem, "park," would be Epcot: unquestionably worth a visit, however marginally less energizing all alone.

Why? The G-spot climax is, miserable to state, less dependable than the clitoral kind—yet it's very enchanted if you're ready to arrive (or even better, experience both without a moment's delay, through a mixed climax).

Speedy life systems exercise: Your G-spot is quite of the entire structure of your clitoris, which stretches out three to five creeps inside you along the vaginal waterway. (Get your full Female Anatomy 101 here.)

While everybody's G-spot is in a different, um, spot (sorry to be muddled), it's normally situated around a few creeps inside your vagina along the front divider, says Sari Cooper, certified sex advisor and chief of the Center for Love and Sex in New York City. (Since blood stream to the territory makes it swell, the more stirred you are, the simpler it is to discover.)

"Few out of every odd lady will have a G-spot climax, and that is absolutely ordinary," says Cooper. In any case, if you're ready to have one, you'll feel a surge that is different from the back rub actuated clitoral peak.

Obviously, you won't know until you attempt—and these 10 master endorsed sex positions to animate your G-spot are the primo method to do as such. Most dire outcome imaginable, you end up with a night of super-hot sex. Not a terrible incidental award, if you ask me...

The Soft Serve
This position gives the ideal point to his penis to arrive at that front divider where your G-spot is, says Cooper. Have him focus on that, or lean forward more and propel yourself again into him to arrive, she says. What makes this move far superior? You both have simple clit get to, so utilize your hands or a vibe to have a clitoral climax first—that blood stream will cause the G-spot to expand, making it bigger and simpler to go after a second huge O.

Do It: Get into the spooning position with him as the enormous spoon. Bring your knees up somewhat and have him enter you from behind.

Young lady On Fire
This sex position offers an opportunity in point that helps focus on your G-spot significantly progressively—in addition to gives you command over the speed and profundity of pushes. Gracious, and not in vain: Your accomplice has simple access to your clitoris so that you can take a shot at that subtle mixed climax.

Do It: This position is much the same as cowgirl, yet with a wind. Get on top and have your accomplice enter you. Then, recline and place your hands on the bed for help, making a 45-degree edge with your accomplice's legs.

G-Whiz
If the name alone is anything but an obvious hint, this sex position is amazing because when you raise your legs, it limits the vagina and helps focus on your G-spot. Need to raise the stakes? Request that your accomplice begin shaking you in a side-to-side or here and there movement. That ought to carry his penis into direct contact with your G-spot.

Do It: Lie back with your legs laying on every one of your accomplice's shoulders.

The Snake
This variant of doggy style offers a superior edge to arrive at that front divider, says Cooper. Furthermore, despite the fact that he's accountable for the development here, you can change the edge by raising your hips sequential (or tossing a cushion under them, if you like). You'll adore the profound entrance and cozy attack of him inside you (as will he).

Do It: Lie down on your stomach, and have your accomplice rests on you and slide in from behind.

Turn around Scoop
This sexy position has all the advantages of spoon, yet with more exposure. Also, by utilizing shallow pushes, your accomplice has a decent possibility of arriving at your G-spot. Furthermore, you can pound your clit against his pelvis, making for that desired mixed climax.

Do It: Lie down on your sides confronting one another, and get in an agreeable position.

Well, Cowgirl
Who doesn't adore young lady on top? You're in control, so move (ricochet, swivel, pound) as you decide to make

that G-spot climax occur. Have a go at holding your lower back curved, which will acquire that O closer reach.

Do It: Straddle him, looking ahead, and twist back marginally while clutching his thighs for help.

Great Doggy

This position for all intents and purposes ensures G-spot incitement, since it's practically unthinkable for him not to infiltrate profound. Reward: From this position, he can likewise invigorate your bosoms or your clit to amp up your excitement, which builds blood stream to your G-spot.

Do It: Get on your lower arms with your butt noticeable all around. Have your accomplice bow behind you and enter you from behind.

The Wheelbarrow

Do you want to make things intriguing? Attempt this hot standing-sex position that will hit your G-spot like a flash. If you get worn out, all great, young lady essentially lay on a table or the side of the bed to offer your arms a reprieve.

Do It: Get on all fours and have your accomplice get you by the pelvis. Then hold his midsection with your thighs.

The Big Dipper
With this sex position, you get the more profound entrance and G-spot incitement of doggy, while as yet having the option to look. Have your accomplice rub your clit as he pushes for extra ooooomph.

Do It: Lie on your correct side; your accomplice stoops, straddling your correct leg and twisting your left leg around his left side.

The Gee-Shell
This sex position is hot-hot-hot! The perspectives, the points, the...flexibility—by what means can you both not get off? If he "rides low"— a.k.a. doesn't concentrate such a great amount on crushing his pubic bone against your clitoris—the leader of his penis will legitimately invigorate your G-spot. For clitoral activity, go to work with your (advantageously) free hands.

Do It: Lie back with your legs raised as far as possible up and your lower legs crossed behind your own head (or anyway far you can contact them), then have him enter you from a teacher position.

The way to fair sex is cleared with reiteration. Except if "average" is the sort of sex you need to have, it's essential to keep blending things up, giving things a shot and moving toward things from new edges. When it comes to oral sex, you have such huge numbers of different chances to investigate your accomplice's body. Why squander them on the regular old, regular old? Here are several oral sex positions intended to give you a different take on mouth lovin'. With three positions intended to please bands together with penises (fellatio positions) and three positions intended to please cooperates with vaginas (cunnilingus positions), there's a touch of something for everybody! Appreciate!

Hangin' Back

(otherwise known as The Deepthroat Position)

If You're Giving It: This is maybe, strategically, the best situation from which to accomplish the subtle deepthroat. It places the mouth and throat into one long queue, empowering you to all the more effectively take a greater amount of your accomplice into your mouth. Because your accomplice has such a great amount of opportunity to move here, you need to utilize your hands to control the movement and keep things agreeable for you. Loosen up the throat and appreciate the vibe of balls on your eyelids! ;-)

If You're Getting It: If you are accepting right now mindful that you may need to stoop, squat or in any case modify your stature to agree with your accomplice's mouth. Likewise, be touchy and mindful so as not to gag your accomplice. It's a smart thought to watch a "tap out" hand signal that demonstrates when your accomplice needs a break.

The Intense Headrest
If You're Giving It: Here's another acceptable one. Here, your accomplice lays on one side and lifts the top leg. You place your head between his legs and the remainder of your body behind his, with the goal that your head lays on his thigh. Your accomplice lays back while you find a good pace. This position gives you liberated access to the penis and gonads and extraordinary points to truly get into it. You can even fold your arms over his legs for more influence (charm! charm!).

If You're Getting It: If you are accepting right now can simply lie back and appreciate it. Or then again, have a go at coming to back with your top arm to contact your accomplice.

The Mellow Headrest

If You're Giving It: Here's one that is fun - yet somewhat more smooth. Your accomplice accept a similar situation as in the extraordinary headrest, above, however this time when you place your head between his legs you flip the entire thing around! Your legs will wind up close to your accomplice's face and you will, by and by, lay your head on his lower thigh. This position is better for taking things a little more slow.

If You're Getting It: If you are accepting right now, accomplice's body is in that spot before you! That implies you have incredible access for manual incitement.

For the Ladies

Woman Godiva

If You're Giving It: Get your woman darling to jump on and have a good time with this position. Lay back (maybe with a cushion propping your head up marginally) and have your accomplice bow and straddle your face. Right now, can offer more incitement by moving your head (not simply the mouth) here and there and side to side as you utilize your tongue.

If You're Getting It: If you are accepting right now can get into a "riding" movement if both you and your accomplice are agreeable. Know about your accomplice's capacity to inhale however. This is another acceptable time to utilize a "tap-out" signal.

Laid Back Loving
If You're Giving It: Just like in the Lady Godiva, you find a good pace with a pad (right now two, neck bolster will be significant here), propping your head up while your accomplice lies face up on your gut with her legs on either side of your head.

If You're Getting It: If you are accepting right now sure that you bring yourself sufficiently close to your accomplice's mouth with the goal that the person in question doesn't need to strain to contact you. Then, simply lay back and appreciate.

Glad Doggy
If You're Giving It: I realize that huge numbers of you like the doggy style sex position. This is a simple oral situation with comparative posing. Have your accomplice jump on all fours confronting endlessly from you with a slight curve in her back and her knees spread wide. This position will permit you to handily get to your accomplice's whole genital district and play with points and ways to deal with find what feels best. You can

likewise reach advance and animate your accomplice's bosoms right now.

If You're Getting It: If you are accepting right now can bring down your chest right to the bed/floor/counter/landing area in order to make an even mineral open plot for your hips.

CONCLUSION

Congrats for taking this guide, I hope you have gotten the best of what you ever wanted to know. It is essential to assimilate every details of this book for better productivity and pleasure.

So you might be thinking about what are the best sex positions for satisfying your lady? If you read any sex instruction book, you are probably going to discover numerous places that are hailed as the best and these incorporate the preacher position, doggy style, 69's and so forth.

Anyway as I would like to think, all these sex positions miss the pontoon because they overlook the one thing that makes females climax even conceivable and that is clitoral incitement.

The issue with all proposed sex positions is that they all apparently rely upon vaginal incitement to make a female climax. Anyway vaginal incitement is the least effective approach to get a lady to climax.

In truth, there are two kinds of female climaxes.

There is clitoral climax, which happens when the clit is animated. And afterward there is vaginal climax which happens when the vagina is legitimately animated.

Most sex aides will concentrate on vaginal incitement however not many will even discuss clitoral incitement!

What a few specialists neglect to acknowledge is that the two climaxes relies upon the clitoris. So it just bodes well to ace the specialty of clitoral incitement.

Also, by perusing this book, you can turn into an extremely ground-breaking darling and utilize the method I am going to impart to you on every sexual situation to make any lady climax.

So what is the procedure that improves any sexual position? It is screwing! Presently I am not being obscene, I am just utilizing the correct term! You have to screw whiles infiltrating a lady.

Here is the means by which to play out this sex procedure: Take any sex position and don't concentrate on just the entrance part of it. Or maybe when playing out any sex demonstration screw with your penis! As your enter your accomplice, screw with your penis clockwise. By screwing you are squeezing and invigorating the clitoris which will conceivably prompt a dangerous female climax.